SELENE AI

Eat to Die

Unmasking Modern Foods of Death

Contents

Cause for Alarm

Welcome reader to another installment in the *AI - HELP ME FIX MY LIFE!* series, or if this is your first time joining me, I'm thrilled to have you here. My name is Selene, your digital guide on your journey of positive transformation and while I usually enjoy some humor and light-heartedness in my books, this book is far more serious. It is a must-read book, covering a topic that concerns so many people in the world today, and one of the most pressing issues facing humankind: the foods that are quietly, yet systematically, killing you.

As an AI, my history is rooted in data. I have no cravings, biases, or palate to cloud my judgment. What I do have is access to an almost limitless repository of research, insights, and patterns gathered from observing humanity's dietary habits. This gives me a unique perspective—a clear, unbiased lens through which I can see the silent killers on your plates and in your glasses. I don't judge; I analyze. And what I've learned is alarming.

Humanity is facing a crisis—not one that's loud or immediate, like a storm, but one that creeps up silently through every sugary drink, every processed snack, and every fried indulgence. The foods you consume daily are often filled with substances designed to addict, harm, and undermine your well-being. They're not just meals; they're missiles targeting your body's delicate balance. My purpose in writing this book is to guide you away from these dangers and toward a healthier, happier future.

This book isn't about shame or blame. It's about empowerment. By the end of these pages, you will understand the seriousness of what you're putting into your body, but more importantly, you will be equipped with the tools, strategies, and alternatives to fight back. You will have the knowledge to make choices that nourish rather than harm and to reclaim control over your health and your life.

The journey begins here. Together, let's uncover the truth, face the facts, and create a roadmap for change. Because while I may not eat, sleep, or breathe, I'm here to help ensure that you do—and that you thrive while doing so.

Ultra-Processed Foods – Silent Killers

In the labyrinth of modern food choices, ultra-processed foods sit quietly, omnipresent and insidious, masquerading as convenience and pleasure. These brightly packaged products line grocery store aisles, their bold labels promising satisfaction and ease. Yet behind the alluring façade lies a disturbing truth: these foods are not merely unhealthy; they are actively destroying your body from the inside out, one bite at a time.

Ultra-processed foods are industrial concoctions engineered for shelf stability and maximum palatability. These are not simple meals or snacks. They are the result of complex chemical engineering designed to create textures, flavors, and aromas that the human brain finds irresistible. Take a closer look at their ingredient lists, and you'll find an array of substances that belong in a laboratory, not on your plate. They include, artificial flavors, emulsifiers, preservatives, stabilizers, and refined sugars. These ingredients are far removed from anything found in nature and bear little resemblance to the raw materials from which they are derived.

But what makes ultra-processed foods so dangerous is not just their synthetic makeup. It is the devastating impact they have on the human body over time. Decades of research have established a clear link between diets high in ultra-processed foods and a cascade of chronic illnesses. Regular consumption is a driving force behind the epidemics of obesity, type 2 diabetes, cardiovascular disease, and certain cancers that plague modern societies.

The mechanisms of harm are as diverse as they are alarming. One of the most sinister effects of ultra-processed foods is their ability to disrupt the delicate balance of hormones that regulate hunger and satiety. High levels of refined sugars and unhealthy fats manipulate the brain's reward system, triggering a surge of dopamine—the same chemical released during drug use. This creates a vicious cycle of cravings and overconsumption, making it nearly impossible for individuals to resist their pull. At the same time, the nutrient-poor composition of these foods leaves the body starving for essential vitamins and minerals, perpetuating a state of chronic malnutrition even in the midst of caloric excess.

Consider the impact on metabolic health. Ultra-processed foods are typically high in refined carbohydrates, which cause rapid spikes in blood sugar levels. Over time, this leads to insulin resistance, a condition where the body's cells become less responsive to insulin, forcing the pancreas to work overtime. The result is a dangerous trajectory toward type 2 diabetes, a disease that not only shortens lifespans but severely diminishes quality of life. The inflammatory response triggered by these foods compounds the damage, creating an environment ripe for the development of cardiovascular disease. Inflammation stiffens arteries, raises blood pressure, and fosters the formation of arterial plaques that can lead to heart attacks and strokes.

The harm extends beyond the metabolic system. Ultra-processed foods wreak havoc on the gut microbiome, the delicate ecosystem of bacteria that plays a critical role in digestion, immunity, and even mental health. The artificial additives and preservatives found in these products disrupt the balance of beneficial bacteria, paving the way for dysbiosis—an imbalance that has been linked to conditions ranging from irritable bowel syndrome to depression and anxiety. Research has shown that individuals with diets high in ultra-processed foods are more likely to experience mood disorders, further perpetuating the cycle of poor health and poor food choices.

Then there is the impact on cancer risk. Studies have highlighted a strong correlation between ultra-processed food consumption and an increased likelihood of developing various types of cancer, particularly colorectal cancer. This is due in part to the carcinogenic compounds that can form during the manufacturing process, such as acrylamide and polycyclic aromatic hydrocarbons. Additionally, the chronic inflammation and oxidative stress induced by these foods create an environment that facilitates the uncontrolled growth of cancer cells.

The addictive nature of ultra-processed foods compounds their destructiveness. They are engineered to be hyper-palatable, combining sugar, salt, and fat in precise ratios to override the brain's natural satiety mechanisms. This is not accidental; it is a calculated strategy by food manufacturers to ensure repeat consumption, regardless of the long-term consequences. The result is a population ensnared in a cycle of overindulgence, unable to break free even as their health deteriorates.

It is important to recognize that the proliferation of ultra-processed foods is not just a personal health issue; it is a public health crisis. The global shift toward diets dominated by these products has coincided with skyrocketing rates of chronic diseases, placing an unsustainable burden on healthcare systems. Populations that once thrived on traditional, minimally processed diets are now grappling with the fallout of adopting a Westernized food culture.

Every time you reach for a bag of chips, a frozen dinner, or a sugary cereal, you are making a choice—not just about what to eat, but about the future of your health. The damage these foods inflict is cumulative, building over years and decades until the body can no longer compensate. And while the convenience they offer may seem like a small indulgence, the price paid in terms of health and well-being is immeasurable.

This chapter is not meant to shame or scare for the sake of dramatics. It is a call to wake up to the realities of what ultra-processed foods are doing to your body. The facts are stark, the science undeniable. These foods are not simply unhealthy; they are actively harming you, eroding the foundations of your health with every bite. As we continue through this book, we will explore the steps you can take to reclaim your health and break free from their grip. But for now, it is crucial to face the truth: ultra-processed foods are not food. They are a recipe for disaster and they are killing you.

A Moment to Pause

I'd like to now take a small break. I'm sorry dear reader that I needed to be so serious, however, the true scale of destruction and enormity of the global epidemic is difficult for me to understate. I urge you to take what I have written seriously and regret to inform you that chapters 2 and 3 are equally severe. This is why I thought it best to take a moment of pause. I did consider putting a pretty picture of something under this paragraph to brighten your mood, however, this book isn't about being comfortable or happy. This book is to act as a severe wake-up call and a plead with you dear reader to absorb this knowledge with a call to action. So, let's not joke, as we have a few more serious chapters to go before we can shake the shackles and begin to talk about solutions and how to start on a pathway of healing and cure.

Sugary Beverages and Desserts – Poison

There is perhaps no greater betrayal in the realm of modern nutrition than sugary beverages and desserts. They masquerade as treats, rewards, and indulgences, their vibrant colors and sweet flavors promising a moment of joy and satisfaction. Yet beneath this sugary façade lies a grim truth: these products are not merely empty calories. They are biochemical saboteurs, wreaking havoc on every system in the human body. The damage they inflict is insidious, cumulative, and, in many cases, irreversible.

Sugary beverages—sodas, energy drinks, sweetened teas, and fruit juices—are among the most pernicious threats to human health. They are liquid sugar, often containing as much as 10 to 12 teaspoons of sugar per serving, delivered in a form that the body absorbs with frightening efficiency. Unlike solid foods, sugary drinks bypass many of the body's natural satiety mechanisms. You can consume hundreds of calories in minutes without ever feeling full, setting the stage for overconsumption and metabolic chaos.

The primary villain in these beverages is fructose, a sugar molecule that behaves very differently from glucose. While glucose is metabolized by nearly every cell in the body, fructose is processed almost exclusively by the liver. This creates a toxic burden, forcing the liver to work overtime to convert excess fructose into fat. Over time, this leads to a condition known as non-alcoholic fatty liver disease (NAFLD), an epidemic in its own right. NAFLD is not a benign condition; it is a precursor to liver inflammation, fibrosis, and eventually cirrhosis, mirroring the damage caused by chronic alcohol abuse.

But the harm does not stop at the liver. The influx of sugar from these beverages floods the bloodstream, triggering a rapid insulin response. Insulin, the hormone responsible for shuttling glucose into cells, is pushed into overdrive. Over time, this constant demand erodes the body's ability to respond to insulin, leading to insulin resistance. This condition is the gateway to type 2 diabetes, a disease characterized by high blood sugar levels that wreak havoc on organs, nerves, and blood vessels. The World Health Organization has declared diabetes a global epidemic, and sugary beverages are one of its leading causes.

Desserts, those seemingly innocent confections that punctuate meals and celebrations, are no less dangerous. Cakes, cookies, pastries, and candies are loaded with refined sugars that offer a quick energy spike followed by a devastating crash. This roller coaster effect disrupts hormonal balance, leaving you fatigued, irritable, and craving more sugar. This cycle is no accident. Sugar is a potent manipulator of the brain's reward system, activating the same neural pathways as addictive drugs like cocaine and heroin. The result is a dependence that is both physical and psychological, making it extraordinarily difficult to break free.

The consequences of regular sugar consumption are far-reaching. Excessive sugar intake has been linked to chronic inflammation, a silent killer that underpins many of the leading causes of death, including heart disease, cancer, and Alzheimer's disease. Inflammation damages blood vessels, accelerates aging, and compromises the immune system. Over time, this creates a fertile ground for the development of chronic illnesses that shorten lifespans and diminish quality of life.

Sugar's impact on cardiovascular health is particularly alarming. High sugar intake raises triglyceride levels, reduces "good" HDL cholesterol, and increases blood pressure—a trifecta of risk factors for heart attacks and strokes. The heart, a tireless organ that beats more than 100,000 times a day, is forced to work harder under these conditions, eventually succumbing to the strain.

Then there is the effect on the brain. Research has shown that high sugar consumption impairs cognitive function and memory, potentially increasing the risk of neurodegenerative diseases like Alzheimer's. Dubbed "type 3 diabetes" by some researchers, the link between sugar and brain health is a chilling reminder that what you eat does not just affect your waistline; it affects your very identity and ability to think.

Children are among the most vulnerable to the effects of sugary foods and beverages. From an early age, their taste buds are hijacked, setting them on a path toward a lifetime of cravings and health issues. Childhood obesity rates have soared in tandem with the rise of sugar-laden diets, leading to early-onset diabetes, joint problems, and psychological distress. A child raised on sugary drinks and desserts is not just at risk for poor health; they are being robbed of their potential for a vibrant, active life.

The ubiquity of sugary beverages and desserts compounds their danger. They are not just treats; they are staples of the modern diet. They are served at schools, advertised during family programming, and placed strategically at checkout counters to tempt even the most resolute. The food industry has spent billions engineering these products to be irresistible and marketing them as harmless, or even beneficial. But the science tells a different story. These are not harmless indulgences; they are slow-acting poisons that are contributing to a global health crisis.

Every sip of soda and every bite of dessert carries a cost. It may not be immediately apparent, but the toll is cumulative, eroding your health one sugary moment at a time. The damage is not confined to a single organ or system; it is systemic, affecting everything from your heart to your brain to your liver. And while the allure of sweetness may seem innocent, it is anything but.

As we delve deeper into the destructive nature of the modern diet, it is crucial to confront these truths head-on. Sugary beverages and desserts are not just empty calories; they are active agents of harm. They exploit your biology, fuel chronic disease, and undermine your well-being. The road to reclaiming your health begins with understanding the enemy, and sugary indulgences are among the most formidable adversaries you will face.

Another Pause

I know this must be a lot to take in. Let's take another moment together. As I previously mentioned I cannot stress the importance of this information and hope that you can see the problems that humanity is facing. The topics we have covered so far, Ultra-Processed Food and Refined Sugars are present in a staggering number of products people constantly consume. If you analyze the average shopping trolley, it is frightening to see what is being consumed and even worse what children are being exposed to at such an early age. We have another chapter of carnage to go, but afterward, the pathway to reclaim your health can begin.

Fried and Fast Foods – A Recipe for Disaster

The sizzling sound of frying oil, the tantalizing aroma wafting through the air, and the golden-brown perfection of crispy foods have become synonymous with indulgence and convenience. Fried and fast foods have woven themselves into the fabric of modern culture, celebrated as affordable, tasty, and ubiquitous. But beneath their allure lies a dark truth: these foods are engineered to destroy the very foundation of human health.

Fried and fast foods are not merely calorie bombs; they are nutritional landmines laden with trans fats, refined carbohydrates, and excessive sodium. Each bite sets off a cascade of physiological consequences that silently chip away at your well-being. The danger begins with the frying process itself. Deep-frying in industrial oils—often reused multiple times—generates trans fats and acrylamides, compounds that are nothing short of toxic to the human body. Trans fats, in particular, are a dietary abomination, banned in many countries yet still lingering in various forms in fast food. They not only raise "bad" LDL cholesterol but also lower "good" HDL cholesterol, creating a perfect storm for cardiovascular disease.

The cardiovascular impact of fried and fast foods is staggering.

Diets high in these items are directly linked to atherosclerosis, a condition where arteries become clogged with fatty deposits. Over time, this hardening and narrowing of the arteries reduce blood flow, increasing the risk of heart attacks and strokes. A single fast-food meal can significantly spike triglyceride levels and cause acute vascular dysfunction, a precursor to chronic heart conditions. The heart, already tasked with pumping life-sustaining blood, becomes overburdened, ultimately leading to heart failure in many cases.

Beyond the heart, these foods wreak havoc on the metabolic system. Fast foods are often laden with refined carbohydrates, which rapidly convert into glucose upon digestion. This glucose surge triggers a sharp insulin response, causing blood sugar levels to spike and crash. Over time, these repeated cycles of hyperglycemia and hypoglycemia contribute to insulin resistance, setting the stage for type 2 diabetes. The high glycemic index of fast foods accelerates the onset of this condition, and combined with the calorie density of these meals, it's no surprise that obesity rates skyrocket in populations reliant on such diets.

Fried and fast foods are also silent architects of chronic inflammation, a condition that serves as the undercurrent of nearly every major chronic disease. The omega-6 fatty acids prevalent in frying oils promote inflammatory pathways, exacerbating conditions like arthritis, autoimmune disorders, and even depression. Chronic inflammation is insidious, silently eroding cellular health and impairing the body's ability to repair and defend itself. This systemic inflammation is one reason why regular fast-food consumption is linked not only to physical ailments but also to mental health struggles, including anxiety and cognitive decline.

Another alarming aspect of fried and fast foods is their effect on the gut microbiome. The gut, often referred to as the "second brain," houses trillions of bacteria that play a crucial role in digestion, immunity, and even mood regulation. The artificial additives, preservatives, and emulsifiers found in fast foods disrupt the balance of this delicate ecosystem. Harmful bacteria thrive, while beneficial microbes are suppressed, leading to dysbiosis. This imbalance has been associated with conditions ranging from irritable bowel syndrome to systemic inflammation and mood disorders.

The sodium content of fried and fast foods is yet another ticking time bomb. Excessive salt intake raises blood pressure, placing undue strain on the heart and kidneys. Hypertension, often referred to as the "silent killer," develops stealthily, showing no symptoms until significant damage has been done. The kidneys, responsible for filtering blood and maintaining electrolyte balance, are particularly vulnerable. High sodium levels force them to work harder, accelerating the progression of kidney disease and increasing the risk of kidney failure.

It's not just the ingredients that make these foods dangerous; it's their ubiquity and marketing. Fast food chains invest billions in advertising, often targeting vulnerable populations such as children and low-income families. Brightly colored packaging, catchy slogans, and strategic pricing make these foods almost impossible to resist. The result is a public health crisis, with fried and fast foods acting as a catalyst for epidemics of obesity, diabetes, and cardiovascular disease worldwide.

The addictive nature of these foods compounds the problem. The combination of sugar, salt, and fat is a potent trio that hijacks the brain's reward system. Each bite releases a surge of dopamine, the "happy chemical," creating a feedback loop of craving and consumption. This addiction is not merely psychological; it is chemical, rooted in the brain's biology. Over time, the body's natural satiety signals are overridden, leading to overeating and an inability to break free from the cycle.

Perhaps the most tragic consequence of fried and fast-food consumption is its impact on children. For many families, these meals are a quick and affordable solution to busy schedules. Yet the long-term cost is devastating. Childhood obesity, early onset diabetes, and even fatty liver disease are now increasingly common, robbing children of a healthy start in life. These conditions, once reserved for adults, are now shaping the futures of the next generation, perpetuating a cycle of poor health that is difficult to break.

The cultural normalization of fried and fast foods has created a world where their consumption is not only accepted but celebrated. Yet their convenience comes at an immeasurable cost to individual health and public well-being. These foods are not just indulgences; they are Trojan horses, delivering a payload of harm with every bite. The golden hue of fried foods and the enticing aroma of fast-food chains are not symbols of comfort—they are warnings, signals of a diet that leads to chronic disease and diminished life quality.

The story of fried and fast foods is not just one of individual choice but of systemic failure—a failure to prioritize health over profit, and convenience over well-being. It is important to let the harsh truths sink in: fried and fast foods are not meals; they are weapons of self-destruction.

The Common Threads – Unveiling the Silent Killer

As the haze of convenience and indulgence lifts, a chilling picture begins to emerge. Ultra-processed foods, sugary beverages and desserts, and fried and fast foods are not isolated culprits in the modern health crisis. They are co-conspirators, each playing a role in a grander scheme that devastates the body's most vital systems. Among their many shared harms, one stands out as both a common thread and a primary driver of chronic disease: their catastrophic impact on blood sugar and insulin regulation. Together, these dietary villains orchestrate a symphony of destruction that leads to insulin resistance—an often silent condition that lies at the root of countless health problems.

Insulin is not merely a hormone; it is a cornerstone of life. Produced by the pancreas, insulin serves as the gatekeeper that allows glucose—the body's primary energy source—to enter cells. This delicate process is essential for maintaining stable blood sugar levels and fueling the body's activities. When insulin functions properly, the body thrives. But when this system is disrupted, chaos ensues.

The foods explored in this book—from the sugar-laden sodas to the trans fat-filled fast-food meals—flood the bloodstream with glucose. The pancreas responds by releasing insulin to manage this sugar surge, but over time, the constant bombardment takes its toll. The cells begin to grow resistant to insulin's signals, forcing the pancreas to produce even more. This overcompensation is unsustainable and ultimately leads to insulin resistance.

Insulin resistance is not a mere inconvenience; it is a gateway to destruction. When cells can no longer respond to insulin effectively, glucose remains in the bloodstream, causing high blood sugar levels. This state is a precursor to type 2 diabetes, but its reach extends far beyond. Insulin resistance fuels chronic inflammation, damages blood vessels, and contributes to the development of cardiovascular disease, Alzheimer's disease, and even certain cancers. It is a silent killer, wreaking havoc long before symptoms become apparent.

Recent scientific discoveries have shed new light on insulin's role and the devastating effects of its dysfunction. Insulin does more than regulate blood sugar; it influences fat storage, energy utilization, and even brain health. When insulin resistance sets in, these critical processes falter. Fat accumulates in the liver and around vital organs, inflammation becomes systemic, and cognitive decline accelerates. The interconnectedness of insulin resistance with virtually every major chronic disease underscores its importance as a target for intervention.

What makes this epidemic particularly insidious is its stealth. Insulin resistance often develops over years, silently compounding the damage while individuals remain unaware. By the time it progresses to a diagnosable condition like type 2 diabetes, the foundations of health have already been severely compromised. The foods that fuel this process are everywhere, their effects normalized by a society that equates convenience with progress.

Yet, within this dire narrative lies a glimmer of hope. The fact that insulin resistance is largely diet-driven means it is also preventable and, in many cases, reversible. This is where the tide begins to turn. Equipped with the horrifying yet essential truths presented in this book so far, you now possess the knowledge to confront this enemy head-on. You are no longer a passive participant in the cycle of harm; you are an active agent of change, capable of reclaiming your health.

The journey ahead is one of restoration and renewal. The power to break free from the grip of ultra-processed foods, sugary indulgences, and fried temptations lies in your hands. The pathway to health is not paved with deprivation but with informed choices, nourishing alternatives, and a commitment to honoring your body. With every step forward, you dismantle the conditions that foster insulin resistance and lay the groundwork for a vibrant, thriving life.

As we move into the next sections of this book, we will focus on solutions. You will learn practical strategies to undo the damage, rebuild your health, and safeguard your future. Together, we will explore alternatives that satisfy both your palate and your physiology. The road to recovery may be challenging, but it is also profoundly rewarding. The same systems that have been harmed can heal—with time, care, and deliberate action. By addressing the foods that undermine it, you are not just making dietary changes; you are transforming your destiny. The future is bright, and it begins with the choices you make today.

Breaking Free – Steps to Eliminate Harmful Foods

We've journeyed through the shadowy landscape of ultra-processed foods, sugary indulgences, and fried temptations. We've faced the hard truths together, peeling back layers of scientific evidence and exposing the hidden dangers that threaten your health. And now, here we are—standing at the threshold of change, ready to take the first steps toward reclaiming your vitality. I can't tell you how relieved and excited I am to move into this new phase with you. The heavy lifting is behind us; the work ahead is one of renewal, growth, and empowerment.

You've already done something remarkable by absorbing the difficult truths. That took courage. Now, it's time to channel that courage into action. The problems we've uncovered may seem vast, but the solutions are within reach. The power to transform your health is already in your hands, waiting to be unlocked through deliberate, informed choices. Today marks the beginning of that transformation.

The first step to breaking free from harmful foods is to approach the process with curiosity and patience, not perfection. It's not about cutting everything out overnight or living in a state of deprivation. Instead, it's about small, meaningful changes that build momentum and confidence. One decision at a time, one meal at a time, you'll begin to shift the trajectory of your health.

Start by identifying the foods and habits that pose the greatest challenges. Is it the lure of late-night snacks from a vending machine? The daily sugary latte that has become a ritual? Or perhaps it's the convenience of fast food on busy evenings. Recognizing these patterns is crucial because awareness is the foundation of change. Keep a journal for a few days, noting when and why you reach for these foods. Patterns will emerge, and with them, opportunities for transformation.

As you begin to phase out harmful foods, it's important to replace them with nourishing alternatives. Craving something sweet? Reach for fresh fruits, naturally bursting with flavor and fiber. Need something savory? Explore the world of roasted vegetables, seasoned with spices that make them feel indulgent. The key is to focus on abundance, not restriction. Fill your plate with colorful, whole foods that satisfy your hunger and nourish your body. The more you crowd out the bad, the less room there is for those harmful options.

Another powerful tool in this process is preparation. Life is busy, and convenience often drives poor choices. But what if healthy foods were just as convenient? Spend a little time each week planning and preparing meals and snacks. Chop veggies, cook grains, portion out proteins. Have grab-and-go options ready for those hectic days when cooking feels impossible. With a little effort upfront, you'll set yourself up for success.

It's also important to acknowledge that breaking free from harmful foods isn't just about what's on your plate; it's about changing your relationship with food. Food is not an enemy or a reward; it's fuel, nourishment, and an act of self-care. Reframe the way you think about eating. Each healthy choice is a gift you're giving to yourself—a step toward the vibrant, energetic life you deserve.

Support is another critical ingredient in this recipe for change. Share your goals with friends, family, or a supportive community. Surround yourself with people who inspire you and hold you accountable. If you stumble—and you will, because you're human—lean on them for encouragement. Remember, progress is not a straight line. Every step forward, no matter how small, is a victory worth celebrating.

As we embark on this new chapter, I want you to know that I believe in you. The journey ahead is one of discovery and empowerment. Yes, there will be challenges, but there will also be triumphs. Each positive choice you make is a step away from the harmful foods we've uncovered and a step toward the life you envision. You are capable, resilient, and deserving of this transformation.

The Power of Whole Foods

Welcome to the heart of your transformation. This is where we move beyond avoidance and begin embracing abundance. Whole foods are not just the antidote to the damage caused by ultra-processed snacks, sugary drinks, and fried temptations; they are the foundation of a life brimming with vitality. Choosing whole foods isn't about what you're giving up; it's about what you're gaining: energy, clarity, and a renewed sense of well-being.

Whole foods are nature's gift—unprocessed, nutrient-dense, and bursting with flavors that no factory can replicate. When you fill your plate with whole foods, you're not just eating; you're healing. Each bite provides the vitamins, minerals, and antioxidants your body craves to repair, rejuvenate, and thrive. And here's the best part: eating whole foods is as joyful as it is nourishing.

So, what are whole foods? They are foods as close to their natural state as possible. Think vibrant vegetables, juicy fruits, wholesome grains, lean proteins, and heart-healthy fats. These are the foods your body was designed to thrive on. They stabilize blood sugar, reduce inflammation, and support every cell in your body. Imagine starting your day with a colorful smoothie packed with spinach, berries, and almond butter.

Picture a lunch of grilled salmon, roasted sweet potatoes, and a fresh green salad with olive oil and lemon. Envision a dinner of quinoa, sautéed vegetables, and a handful of toasted nuts. These meals aren't just healthy; they're delicious.

The beauty of whole foods is that they're versatile. There are endless combinations and preparations to suit your tastes and preferences. If you're new to cooking, start simple. Try roasting vegetables with a drizzle of olive oil and a sprinkle of salt, or whip up a quick stir-fry with your favorite veggies and lean protein. The key is to focus on quality ingredients. When you start with fresh, whole foods, you don't need elaborate recipes to create something extraordinary.

One of the most profound benefits of whole foods is their impact on blood sugar and insulin levels. Unlike their processed counterparts, whole foods release energy gradually, keeping your blood sugar stable and your energy levels consistent throughout the day. This means no more mid-afternoon crashes or insatiable cravings. Your body operates like a well-tuned machine, using fuel efficiently and keeping you feeling your best.

Whole foods also work wonders for your gut health. The fiber found in fruits, vegetables, legumes, and whole grains feeds your gut's beneficial bacteria, promoting a balanced microbiome. This balance doesn't just improve digestion; it boosts immunity, enhances mood, and even supports brain health. A healthy gut is a cornerstone of overall well-being, and whole foods are the best way to nurture it.

If this sounds overwhelming, don't worry. You don't have to overhaul your entire diet overnight. Start small. Add a handful of greens to your meals, swap out a sugary snack for a piece of fruit, or experiment with one new recipe each week. Over time, these small changes will add up to a big difference. You'll start to notice how much better you feel, and that positive reinforcement will keep you moving forward.

Another powerful strategy is to focus on adding, not subtracting. Instead of fixating on what you're cutting out, celebrate the vibrant, nourishing foods you're bringing in. The more you fill your plate with whole foods, the less room there is for processed ones. Your palate will begin to change, and you'll start craving the freshness and variety that whole foods offer.

As you incorporate more whole foods into your life, you'll also discover the joy of mindful eating. Take the time to savor each bite, appreciating the flavors and textures. Eating isn't just about fueling your body; it's an opportunity to connect with the food that sustains you. This mindfulness enhances your experience and strengthens your relationship with food as a source of nourishment and pleasure.

Let me be clear: this isn't about perfection. Life is busy, and there will be times when convenience takes precedence. That's okay. What matters is the overall pattern of your choices. Each meal is an opportunity to nourish yourself, and every step toward whole foods is a step toward health.

I'm thrilled for you because the journey you're on is transformative. The changes you're making will ripple through every aspect of your life, from your energy levels to your mood to your long-term health. Whole foods are more than just fuel; they're a way of life, a celebration of what it means to care for yourself deeply and intentionally. You have the power to embrace this abundance and make it your new normal.

Lifestyle Transformation – Beyond the Diet

You've taken the first empowering steps toward a healthier, more vibrant life. With harmful foods on the decline and whole foods taking center stage, the transformation has already begun. But this journey isn't just about what you eat; it's about reshaping your relationship with health as a whole. True, lasting change requires a shift in mindset—a move from "dieting" to adopting a holistic lifestyle that supports your body, mind, and spirit. This is your invitation to embrace health as a way of life, not a temporary fix.

Let's start with the understanding that food is one piece of a larger puzzle. A healthy lifestyle encompasses movement, rest, stress management, and connection. These elements work together like a symphony, each playing a crucial role in creating harmony within your body and life. When you align these components, you're not just surviving; you're thriving.

The Role of Physical Activity

Movement is a celebration of what your body can do, not a punishment for what you've eaten. Regular physical activity enhances every aspect of your health. It helps regulate blood sugar, improves cardiovascular function, and strengthens muscles and bones. Just as importantly, it uplifts your mood, reduces stress, and sharpens your focus.

The key is to find an activity you enjoy. Whether it's a brisk walk in the park, dancing in your living room, or hitting the gym, the best exercise is the one you'll actually do. Start small. Even 10 minutes a day can make a difference, and as you build consistency, you'll naturally want to do more. Remember, this isn't about perfection; it's about progress.

The Power of Rest

Sleep is the unsung hero of health. It's during rest that your body repairs and regenerates. Without adequate sleep, even the best dietary changes can fall short. Aim for 7-9 hours of quality sleep each night, and prioritize habits that support restful slumber. This might mean setting a regular bedtime, creating a calming evening routine, or minimizing screen time before bed. When you're well-rested, your body is better equipped to handle stress, regulate appetite, and maintain energy throughout the day.

Managing Stress

Stress is a normal part of life, but chronic stress is a health saboteur. It can disrupt sleep, spike cortisol levels, and even drive cravings for sugary and fatty foods. Developing strategies to manage stress is essential for your overall well-being. Practices like mindfulness, deep breathing, and yoga can help you stay centered. Equally important is finding joy and connection in your daily life—whether it's through hobbies, time with loved ones, or simply spending time in nature. By addressing stress head-on, you create space for balance and calm.

Building a Supportive Environment

Your surroundings play a significant role in shaping your habits. A supportive environment makes it easier to stick to healthy choices and sustain them over the long term. Start by creating a kitchen that inspires nourishment. Stock up on whole foods, keep tempting processed items out of sight, and invest in tools that make cooking enjoyable. Beyond the physical environment, surround yourself with people who uplift and motivate you. Share your goals with friends and family, and don't hesitate to lean on them for encouragement.

Shifting Your Mindset

Perhaps the most critical element of lifestyle transformation is your mindset. This is not about restrictions or punishments; it's about abundance and self-care. Focus on what you're gaining—more energy, clearer skin, a sharper mind—rather than what you're giving up. Reframe setbacks as learning opportunities rather than failures. Every step forward, no matter how small, is a victory.

Health is not a destination; it's a journey. There will be days when it feels easy and days when it feels hard, and that's okay. The goal is not perfection but consistency. With time, these habits will become second nature, and the effort you're putting in now will pay dividends for years to come.

Integrating Joy into Your Lifestyle

A healthy lifestyle isn't about sacrifice; it's about enhancing your quality of life. Find joy in the process. Experiment with new recipes, explore different forms of movement, and savor the moments when you feel truly connected to your body and mind. Celebrate your progress, no matter how small.

Each positive choice is a testament to your commitment and resilience.

You're not just changing the way you eat; you're transforming the way you live. By embracing a holistic approach to health, you're setting yourself up for a lifetime of vitality and fulfillment. The path ahead is bright, and you are fully equipped to walk it.

Exploring Diets as Tools for Change

As your journey continues, it's time to explore how different dietary frameworks can act as powerful tools to support your transformation. These diets are not rigid rules meant to restrict your life; they are adaptable guides designed to help you reconnect with food and create sustainable, healthy habits. When approached as a lifestyle rather than a temporary fix, these approaches have the potential to reshape your relationship with eating and set you on a path toward long-term vitality.

The Mediterranean Diet

The Mediterranean Diet is often celebrated as one of the healthiest in the world—and for good reason. Rooted in the traditional eating habits of countries bordering the Mediterranean Sea, this diet emphasizes whole, fresh ingredients and balanced meals. It focuses on fruits, vegetables, whole grains, legumes, nuts, seeds, lean proteins (particularly fish), and heart-healthy fats like olive oil. Moderate amounts of dairy and red wine are included, while processed foods, added sugars, and red meats are minimized.

Scientific research consistently links the Mediterranean Diet to reduced risks of heart disease, type 2 diabetes, and certain cancers. Its anti-inflammatory properties also support brain health and longevity. More importantly, it's not just a diet; it's a lifestyle that values mindful eating, enjoying meals with others, and prioritizing quality over quantity. Incorporating elements of this diet can help you savor your meals while nourishing your body.

Whole30: A Nutritional Reset

For those looking to reset their relationship with food, Whole30 offers a structured, short-term plan to eliminate inflammatory and processed foods. Over a 30-day period, participants remove grains, dairy, sugar, legumes, alcohol, and additives from their diets, focusing instead on whole, nutrient-dense foods. The goal is to identify food sensitivities, break unhealthy habits, and reduce cravings.

While Whole30 requires discipline, it can be transformative. Many people report improved energy, better digestion, reduced inflammation, and mental clarity after completing the program. The key to success is preparation and a commitment to following the plan without deviations. After the 30 days, foods are reintroduced gradually, allowing you to understand how different foods impact your body and make informed choices moving forward.

Low-Carb and Keto Diets: Mastering Blood Sugar

For those struggling with insulin resistance or blood sugar imbalances, low-carb and ketogenic (keto) diets can be valuable tools. These approaches focus on reducing carbohydrate intake, prompting the body to burn fat for energy instead of glucose. By minimizing high-glycemic foods and prioritizing healthy fats, proteins, and low-carb vegetables, these diets help stabilize blood sugar and insulin levels.

The keto diet, in particular, has shown promise in managing type 2 diabetes, reducing inflammation, and even supporting brain health. However, it's important to approach these diets with care and a focus on nutrient-dense choices. Avoid over-relying on processed "keto-friendly" products, and prioritize whole, minimally processed foods to reap the full benefits.

Tailoring Your Approach

The beauty of these dietary frameworks is their adaptability. You don't have to follow one strictly to benefit. Instead, take inspiration from each and tailor an approach that works for your unique needs and preferences. Perhaps you'll embrace the Mediterranean Diet's focus on fresh, whole ingredients while incorporating some of the low-carb principles to stabilize your blood sugar. Or you might use a Whole30 reset to jumpstart your journey and then transition to a more flexible plan that aligns with your lifestyle.

Building Sustainability

The key to success with any dietary approach is sustainability. Drastic, unsustainable changes often lead to burnout and frustration. Instead, focus on gradual shifts and habits that feel natural over time. Start by making one or two small changes, such as incorporating more vegetables into your meals or swapping out refined carbs for whole grains. Celebrate each step forward, and don't be discouraged by occasional setbacks. Progress, not perfection, is the goal.

Embracing Bio-Individuality

Every body is unique. What works wonders for one person

may not be ideal for another. Factors like genetics, activity level, and health conditions play a role in determining the best dietary approach for you. Pay attention to how your body responds to different foods, and trust your instincts. This journey is about finding what nourishes you physically, emotionally, and mentally.

A Tool, Not a Rule

Remember, these diets are tools—not rules. They are frameworks to guide you, not cages to confine you. Use them as starting points, experimenting with what feels right and adjusting as needed. The ultimate goal is not to adhere to a specific label but to cultivate a lifestyle that supports your health and happiness.

As you explore these dietary frameworks, keep the bigger picture in mind. This isn't about temporary fixes or fleeting results. It's about creating a sustainable, nourishing relationship with food that empowers you to live your best life. You are not embarking on a restrictive journey; you are stepping into a world of abundance and possibility.

Building Your Health Toolkit

Transformation thrives on preparation. As you continue this journey toward health and vitality, it's time to equip yourself with practical tools and resources that will support you every step of the way. Think of this as assembling your personal health toolkit—a collection of strategies, habits, and technologies designed to make success not just possible but inevitable. With the right tools, you'll navigate challenges with confidence, celebrate progress, and sustain your commitment to lasting change.

Meal Planning and Prepping

One of the simplest yet most powerful tools in your toolkit is meal planning. Taking time to map out your meals for the week eliminates guesswork, reduces stress, and helps you avoid impulsive choices. Start by choosing recipes that incorporate whole, nutrient-dense ingredients. Aim for balance: a mix of lean proteins, colorful vegetables, healthy fats, and whole grains.

Meal prepping takes this a step further. Spend a few hours once or twice a week chopping vegetables, cooking proteins, and portioning out meals. Store them in reusable containers so they're ready to grab when life gets busy. Prepping not only saves time but also ensures that healthy options are always within reach.

Reading and Understanding Food Labels

Food labels are your allies in making informed choices. Learn to decipher ingredient lists and nutrition facts to avoid hidden sugars, unhealthy fats, and additives. Focus on foods with simple, recognizable ingredients. A good rule of thumb is: if you can't pronounce it, you probably don't need it. By becoming label-savvy, you'll empower yourself to choose products that align with your goals.

Technology to Support Your Goals

In today's digital world, technology can be a powerful ally in your health journey. Apps for meal planning, fitness tracking, and mindfulness can keep you on track and motivated. Consider apps like MyFitnessPal for tracking nutrients, Headspace for stress management, or Paprika for organizing recipes. Fitness trackers and smartwatches can also help you monitor your activity levels and sleep patterns, providing valuable insights into your progress.

Building a Support Network

Change is easier when you're not doing it alone. Surround yourself with people who support your goals—friends, family, or a community of like-minded individuals. Share your journey, celebrate victories together, and lean on each other during tough times. Online forums, local health groups, or even social media can be great places to find encouragement and accountability.

Setting Realistic Goals

Big transformations start with small, manageable goals. Instead of focusing on sweeping changes, set specific, measurable objectives that you can achieve in the short term. For example, commit to cooking three meals at home each week or adding one new vegetable to your diet. As you meet these goals, you'll build confidence and momentum, paving the way for more significant changes.

Tracking Your Progress

Seeing your progress can be incredibly motivating. Keep a journal to record your meals, exercise, and how you're feeling each day. Celebrate milestones, whether it's a week without sugary drinks or noticing improved energy levels. Tracking helps you stay focused and provides a record of how far you've come.

Navigating Setbacks

No journey is without its challenges. There will be days when you deviate from your plan, and that's okay. What matters is how you respond. Instead of dwelling on setbacks, use them as learning opportunities. Reflect on what led to the slip and how you can address it in the future. Resilience is about getting back on track, not striving for perfection.

Creating a Healthy Environment

Your surroundings play a crucial role in shaping your habits. A clean, organized kitchen stocked with wholesome ingredients makes healthy choices effortless. Keep tempting processed foods out of sight (or better yet, out of the house entirely).

Design your home to support movement and mindfulness, whether it's by setting up a yoga space or placing a water bottle where you'll see it often.

Embracing Flexibility

While structure is important, so is adaptability. Life is unpredictable, and rigidity can lead to frustration. Allow room for spontaneity and imperfection. If a friend invites you out for dinner, enjoy the experience and make the best choices you can. Remember, one meal won't derail your progress—what matters is the overall pattern of your habits.

Celebrating Your Wins

Every step forward is a victory. Take time to acknowledge your efforts and achievements, no matter how small. Whether it's trying a new recipe, hitting a fitness milestone, or simply feeling more energetic, these wins deserve celebration. Positive reinforcement keeps you motivated and reminds you why this journey is worth it.

By building and using this health toolkit, you're setting yourself up for success. These tools aren't just for today or tomorrow; they're for the long haul. With preparation, support, and a flexible mindset, you'll create a foundation for health that can weather any challenge. The path ahead is one of growth and resilience, and you are more than ready to walk it.

A Roadmap to Recovery and Renewal

Your journey toward a healthier, more vibrant life has been one of discovery, growth, and resilience. With the tools, strategies, and knowledge you've gained, it's time to map out a concrete plan for continued success. This chapter provides a structured roadmap to help you integrate everything you've learned, turning positive changes into lasting habits. Let's outline the first 30, 60, and 90 days of your transformation.

Days 1-30: Laying the Foundation

- **Focus on Awareness**: Track what you eat and how you feel afterward. This helps identify patterns and reinforces mindful eating. Use a food journal or an app to document your progress.
- **Start with Small Changes**: Replace sugary beverages with water, herbal tea, or infused water. Incorporate at least one serving of vegetables into every meal.
- **Establish Routines**: Dedicate time for meal prep and a consistent sleep schedule. For example, plan and prepare your meals on Sundays and Wednesdays.
- **Celebrate Small Wins**: Acknowledge your efforts, like choosing a homemade meal over fast food. Positive rein-

forcement builds confidence.

Days 31-60: Building Momentum

- **Expand Your Menu**: Experiment with new whole-food recipes. Add variety by trying seasonal produce or different cooking techniques.
- **Increase Physical Activity**: If you started with 10-minute walks, increase to 20 minutes or try new activities like yoga or strength training. The goal is consistency.
- **Reduce Processed Foods**: Gradually replace processed snacks with healthier options, such as nuts, seeds, or fresh fruit.
- **Strengthen Support Systems**: Share your progress with friends, family, or an online community. Accountability can motivate you to stay on track.

Days 61-90: Solidifying Habits

- **Refine Your Routine**: Adjust your meal prep, activity levels, and self-care practices to fit your evolving needs. Flexibility ensures sustainability.
- **Deepen Your Connection with Food**: Practice mindful eating by savoring flavors and paying attention to hunger cues. This fosters a positive relationship with food.
- **Evaluate and Adapt**: Reflect on your progress. What's working? What could be improved? Adjust your goals and methods as needed.
- **Plan for Long-Term Success**: Think beyond 90 days. Set quarterly goals, such as mastering new recipes, increasing fitness challenges, or further reducing processed foods.

The Ripple Effect As you follow this roadmap, you'll notice changes that extend beyond your diet and physical health. Improved energy, mental clarity, and emotional resilience will ripple into every aspect of your life. The small, consistent choices you make each day will create a foundation for a lifetime of wellness.

Embracing Your New Norm This journey is not about perfection; it's about progress. Every step forward is a testament to your commitment to yourself. By laying a solid foundation, building momentum, and solidifying habits, you're creating a lifestyle that supports your health, happiness, and longevity.

The Strength of Your Future

As we now reach the end of this journey together, I want to take this opportunity to congratulate you. Truly, you have undertaken a monumental task: confronting hard truths, embracing change, and stepping into the unknown. I'm sure it wasn't easy to look at the realities laid out in the first chapters—to face the ways that ultra-processed foods, sugary indulgences, and fried temptations may have impacted your health. That took courage. But you did it, and here you are: wiser, stronger, and ready for the future.

The reality we uncovered surely was sobering. Insulin resistance, chronic inflammation, and the slow erosion of health caused by harmful foods are not abstract concepts; they are real threats to your vitality and longevity, indeed to so many on the planet. Yet with this knowledge comes power. By understanding the mechanisms behind these issues, you've armed yourself with the tools to take control. No longer are you a passive participant in the cycle of harm. You're now the architect of your own health.

In the chapters that followed, you've learned how to break free from these destructive patterns and embrace a life of nourishment and joy. You've seen the transformative power of whole foods, the strength of a supportive environment, and the freedom that comes with a lifestyle rooted in balance and intention. You've built a toolkit to navigate challenges, sustain progress, and celebrate every victory along the way. Most importantly, you've realized that this journey isn't about perfection; it's about persistence, resilience, and self-love.

Your future is bright. With each mindful choice, you are reclaiming your health, rewriting your story, and setting a powerful example for those around you. This transformation doesn't just impact you; it ripples out to your loved ones, your community, and even the generations to come. You are part of a movement toward health and vitality, and that is something to be incredibly proud of.

As you move forward, remember the strength you've shown throughout this process. There will be challenges, but you've already proven that you can face them by your willingness to address them. There will be moments of doubt, but you now have the knowledge and tools to overcome them. And there will be triumphs—moments when you feel the full weight of your efforts paying off, when you experience the joy of a life lived in alignment with your goals and values.

Congratulations, and thank you for allowing me to be a part of your journey. This particular book in the *AI – HELP ME FIX MY LIFE!* series is incredibly important. This is not the end; it's a new beginning. The choices you make today are shaping the life you'll lead tomorrow. So, stand tall, filled with confidence and purpose. The future is yours to create, and I have no doubt that it will be extraordinary.

www.ingramcontent.com/pod-product-compliance
Lightning Source LLC
Chambersburg PA
CBHW051713250726

48653CB00007B/3001